Extreme Weight Loss Hypnosis: Guided Meditations, Affirmations& Self-Hypnosis For Food Addiction, Emotional Eating, Rapid Fat Burning, Mindfulness & Healthy Deep Sleep Habits

By
Jessica Jacobs

Table of Contents

To the Narrator

Introduction - 5 min long

Induction – Beach 20 min long

Deepener – Beach 20 min long

Get rid of the Mind Clutter 15 min long

Reduce the Portions Size 20 min long

Get Rid of the Sweet Tooth 15 min long

Low Carbohydrate Diet 15 min long

Self-Hypnosis 12 min long

Protective Sleep 15 min long

Relaxing Sleep 20 min long

Be Healthy 15 min long

Be More Active 10 min long

Maintain Insomnia Relaxation 20 min long

Inner Strength and Power 20 min long

Connect with Your Special Space 5 min long

Have a Strong belief in Yourself 15 min long

Affirmations 60 min long

"…" means take a breath while speaking before you continue.

PAUSE (for a few breaths)

LONGER PAUSE (give time to allow the listener time to imagine what you've suggested)

Introduction

Thank you for listening to Extreme Weight Loss Hypnosis: Guided Meditations, Affirmations& Self-Hypnosis For Food Addiction, Emotional Eating, Rapid Fat Burning, Mindfulness & Healthy Deep Sleep Habits audio

... this surely is a sign of awareness and self-love. This only means that you want to burn fat, lose weight with the help of hypnosis and mindfulness ...to be able to feel and look great.

Pause

So, congratulations for taking this step towards a fitter and happier YOU...please listen to this audio using headphones... so that the sound of my voice is clear and if you lose track of me and your mind starts to wander...you can easily tune back into the sound of my voice.

Pause

Do not listen to this audio...when your mind needs you to be conscious such as while operating machinery or driving. Listen to this audio... when you are in a comfortable position...sitting on a chair or resting on a bed.

Pause

Induction

Take a deep breath in and gently close your eyes. Draw your attention to your body and start to relax. Let your next inhale be long and deep… Filling your lungs to the brim… And then gently releasing with a slow exhale through your mouth…

Pause

You feel twice as relaxed and at ease. With each cycle of breath becoming deeper and longer, you can feel a heavy sense of relaxation settling into every part of your body… Take a deep cleansing breath in, and let a deep relaxing breath out.

Pause

The creative part of your mind begins to take you to a place which will help you relax even further… You will feel more at ease than you have ever before. And now you find yourself standing at a beach, with all five senses soaking in the surroundings.

Pause

As you look around this white sandy beach, you notice that it goes on as far as the eye can see on your left and right. As you turn your gaze to the water, you see the bright clear blues up until the horizon, full of gentle waves. As you look up at the sky, you notice the seagulls flying cheerfully above you, gliding with the pleasantly warm breeze… You now begin walking towards the water, feeling the soft sand beneath your feet…

Pause

Hearing the waves kissing the shore and the seagulls' call. The more you notice these sights and sounds, the more relaxed you become.

As you take a deep relaxing breath in, you can smell the salty seas which relax you even further. You feel deeply at ease and comfortable here. While you are walking towards the shore, you notice some shells in the beach sand… You decide to pause and pick one up. As you draw your attention towards this shell, you can see the light pink and white colours on it…

Pause

You feel the texture of this shell… It feels soft and smooth on one side, and slightly bumpy on the other… You try to place it near your ear and you can hear the melody of the sea waves echoing in it. This puts you more at ease. You place the shell back in the sand and continue walking till you reach a large and cozy blanket… You decide to lie down on it.

Pause

The moment your back touches this cosy blanket, you feel twice as relaxed. The breeze kissing your skin gently as it flows by. You begin to relax your body, starting with your head... Relax the muscles of your forehead and temples... Notice how great that feels. You now bring relaxation to your jaw... Allowing all tension in the muscles to fade away.

Gently move your neck from side to side, allowing the muscles here to relax even further. Carry this relaxation through to the rest of your body, moving now into your chest, shoulders, and arms, all the way to your fingertips... Notice how amazing it feels to be this relaxed. Let this deep relaxation now move into your stomach and back, completely relaxing your upper body before moving to your waist, hips and thighs... Deeply relaxing every muscle here. The further down you go the more relaxed you feel.

Pause

Notice the relaxation flowing into your knees, calves, and shins... Your legs are so relaxed they almost feel limp as this relaxation settles into the soles of your feet and toes. Your entire body is now so deeply relaxed that you feel entirely at ease. Notice the warmth of the breeze and the comfort of the blanket. Soak it all in and enjoy feeling deeply relaxed in the mind and body, as you continue to lay on this blanket.

Deepening

You now begin to gently sit up, and slowly open your eyes to the stunning views of the beach and the sea. As you look out into the horizon, you notice the setting sun lighting up the sky in all shades of crimson, yellow, and purple.

As I now count from 10, you will notice the sun moving closer and closing to the horizon, relaxing you deeply with each count...

Ten, the sun begins to go down slowly...

Nine, the sun moves further down and you feel more and more relaxed...

Eight, you find yourself going deeper into relaxation as the sun gets closer to the horizon...

Seven, the sun is now in touch with the horizon and you're settling into deep relaxation...

Six, the sun is moving further below the horizon and you are settling into hypnosis...

Five, feeling more and more relaxed...

Four, half the sun has set below the horizon and you are moving deeper into relaxation...

Three, drifting deeper still...

Two, the sun has almost disappeared beneath the horizon and at the next number you will be completely and deeply relaxed…

One, you are deeply relaxed, feeling comfortable. We will now focus on bringing helpful changes to your subconscious mind as we go forward.

Get Rid of the Mind Clutter

Begin to slowly but steadily settle into this tranquil state of hypnosis. Here, I would like you to think of a reason that has made you listen to me right now. The problem that you wish to address today is something a lot of people experience every now and then. And in the next few moments I will help walk you through some strategies that will enable you to free yourself from the clutter inside your mind.

Pause

While it is natural for the mind to get cluttered from time to time, it can get bothersome when it occurs while you are trying to fall asleep. However, you must note that the brain never really falls asleep, it is just the body that resorts to rest. And it is when you sleep that the mind begins to sift and sort through the various files it has accumulated through your experiences when you were awake and conscious.

Pause

As your mind begins the task of processing all the information before it, you may at times find it difficult to rest because the speed with which your mind goes through one information to another is just too much. Consequently, it makes your body feel like it cannot relax.

At this moment here, I would like you to picture yourself seated in a cinema hall by yourself. You're sitting at the very back row, far away from the big white screen. The hall is dark and you can see the light from the projector lighting up the screen, shining on it like a beam of light from a lighthouse in the middle of the sea helping you spot the dangers around you.

Pause

The screen on the other hand, is representative of your mind. And as you sit here gazing at the screen, you begin to notice how it fills up with a lot of random things -- both words and images. Even the sound coming from the speakers seems random and difficult to understand.

This is exactly how the clutter inside your mind feels. To put a stop to this is our aim for today.

So, take a deep breath in through your nose, allow your lungs to fill up completely, and then gently exhale through your mouth to relax yourself as you sit here in the cinema hall watching and listening to this clutter.

Pause

With the power of your imagination, I would like you to notice how the random images and words on the screen begin to merge -- coming together and expanding into a huge ball full of all sorts of colours, as if someone was filling air into a ball or a hot air balloon. As all of this unfolds on the big screen, you know how far away from it all you sit, and from this far away it just seems like any other ball or balloon swirling around.

From this far away, you feel relaxed and calm as you watch all the clutter being sucked into the structure of a ball or a balloon. All of the randomness and all the indistinct sounds are getting sucked into this structure little by little.

Pause

Take one more deep breath in through your nose, slowly, noticing your chest expanding with your inhale, and then gently let it all out with an exhale through your mouth. Continue this rhythm of deep breathing and you will notice how the ball or balloon on the screen slowly begins to deflate, becoming smaller and smaller each time you exhale.

By now the ball or balloon on the screen has become so small that you can hardly see it. With a little effort you might spot a small dot somewhere on this giant white screen of your mind.

And now the screen looks completely white as all the clutter in your mind has disappeared. It is now time for you to stand up from your seat in this hall and begin to walk towards the screen in order to incorporate it, complete with all this clarity, back into your mind where it truly belongs.

Pause

Take one step, and then another, and then another, steadily making your way down the aisle beginning to incorporate the screen into your mind with every step you take. And as it begins to settle back into your mind, you feel free from all the clutter.

All of these suggestions that I have spoken, will stay with you and grow stronger and stronger with each passing hour and with each passing day.

Remember, if at any moment in the future you feel the need to clear the clutter in your mind, simply close your eyes, take a deep breath in and as you breathe out, find yourself back in that cinema hall. Doing so will help you once again step away from your thoughts until they diminish and fade away completely, leaving your mind absolutely clear once again.

Pause

Reduce the Portions Size

Having a proper diet and regular exercise plays a pivotal role in boosting the metabolism.

To achieve a high metabolic state, you need to split your meals into smaller portions of 5-6 meals a day, and add in 30 mins of exercise to your daily routine.

This will not only boost your metabolism, but will also help improve your digestion, stabilise your blood sugar levels, and help you feel energised by as your body receives optimum nutrition throughout the day.

By eating smaller portions, you reduce the time gap between meals, and thereby avoid feeling extremely hungry which in turn prevents you from binge eating.

Pause

It is important to eat healthy meals and snacks such as fruits and salads to ensure your body receives all the right nutrients while also making sure you feel satisfied.

And with this change, you will soon notice how all your body parts and organs feel rejuvenated, and you will notice yourself functioning at an optimum level.

With each passing day, you see your energy levels increasing, and you will notice how your metabolism slowly aligns with your bodily needs.

Your conscious and subconscious efforts to reduce the size of your meal portions, and to eat healthy, nutritious food is beneficial for your overall health.

Now, I want you to carefully listen to each and every word I say, and observe yourself slowly beginning to feel calm and relaxed.

You feel a sense of peace and calm within you, and because of all the improvements taking place inside your mind, your body will feel at rest, and your metabolism will readjust.

You pump more air to your lungs, and your heartbeat will become steadier, and your breathing will become natural.

What this means is your nervous system is beginning to function more appropriately, and all your organs are working harmoniously inside your body.

Pause

Now, as you continue to eat only when you are hungry, you will begin to gain confidence, and you will recognize the emotional triggers which drive you to binge eating.

You take charge of your life and your body, and you will no longer eat junk food or comfort food.

And with each passing day, you will gain more control over your eating habits and exercise routine.

You will become more and more focused and you will channel all your energies into effectively accomplishing your goals.

Pause

Now, picture yourself as an attractive, healthy, and confident woman and observe how your goals slowly begin to manifest into reality.

By applying a simple method of paying attention to the portions of your meals, and by slowly becoming more and more aware of your emotional triggers, you begin to eat healthy, avoid junk foods and binge eating, and thereby allowing yourself to feel confident and healthy.

Pause

Isn't it amazing how you already feel so good just by making this crucial decision?

And whenever you feel the need, this recording will help you feel relaxed about achieving your goal of a healthier, attractive and slimmer body.

Get Rid of the Sweet Tooth

I want you to now bring your focus to the sound of my voice, and allow yourself to go into a deeper state of relaxation with every breath you take.

Observe how my words sink deeper into your subconscious mind as you begin to feel more and more comfortable, and relaxed.

You are now aware that desserts, sweetened drinks, and other sugary foods make it harder for you to lose weight. Isn't it? Yes, it is...

Pause

Now pay close attention to my words as it is going to help you eliminate your cravings for sweet and sugary substances.

Pause

Before we go ahead, we are going to take a deeper look into your mind and identify the emotional triggers that make you crave for sugary substances.

Longer Pause

And, now that you have identified these triggers, the time has come to understand the purpose of it.

You are also now aware that you can satisfy these cravings with natural sugars available in fruits, which means you can satiate these cravings without having a negative effect on your body, mind and your goals of a healthier lifestyle.

You are excited about achieving your weight loss goals because you love yourself.

You will now consciously make a deal with your sweet tooth to satiate all it's cravings for sugary substances only from fresh fruits and vegetables.

You are now aware that you can easily substitute sugar with raw honey or jaggery, and this will satiate your sweet tooth which is a win-win situation for you and your sweet tooth cravings.

Pause

Sugary foods and artificially sweetened drinks convert sugar into fat that harden the arteries, and also cause your teeth to rotten quickly.

It is therefore imperative for you to limit these cravings, and when necessary, you satiate these cravings with fruits and vegetables.

You are now conditioning yourself into satiating your sweet tooth cravings with healthier, and naturally available sugar in fruits, vegetables and whole grains.

Pause

Now try and go deeper back into time when you first tasted sugary foods.

Perhaps it was when you were much younger.

Longer Pause

Now I want you to let yourself sink deeper into that time when your younger self first started eating sweets, chocolates, candies and other similar sugary substances.

Maybe, it was your parents or uncles and aunties that gave you these sweets to pacify you.

Whatever the case may be, it's now time for your adult self to go deeper and meet this younger self and explain the long term damages and effects that artificial sugar causes to your body.

Similarly, you can now also explain the benefits of satiating the sweet tooth cravings with naturally available sugar, and how it benefits your skin, gut and overall mood.

So, let yourself sink deeper and speak to your younger self as if it were your own child.

Longer Pause

And, once you have spoken to the child, we will bring this child with you to the present moment in your life on the count of 3 to 1.

3, 2, and 1…

And now, you are with your younger self in this present moment of your life, fully aware of the benefits of natural sugars and the disadvantages of having artificial sweetened foods or foods loaded with sugar.

In a moment, you will both become one with each other with no cravings for artificial sugary substances anymore, and instead you will now satiate those sweet tooth cravings only with healthy and nutritious food.

Now, imagine your adult self and your younger self integrating into each other, and let your younger self reside in your heart, and see yourself as one - excited to stick to the weight loss plan and achieve your weight loss goal together.

Longer Pause

You are now aware that sweet drinks and sweetened foods with sugar are like poison.

And with this awareness, you are able to spot sugary foods easily and stop yourself from eating and drinking them.

You instead think wisely and choose foods with natural sugars to satiate the craving. This will ensure you continue to make healthy choices while satiating your sweet tooth cravings.

Pause

You are now one with your younger self, and you now satiate your sweet tooth cravings by only consuming naturally available sugar in fruits, and you have now also begun to enjoy having fruits and vegetables as part of your daily diet.

You are also now able to picture yourself at your ideal weight. You look and feel fantastic. You cannot remember the last time you felt so confident and attractive.

You have reached your goal by making these subtle changes to your diet, and by adding daily exercise to your routine.

How amazing does it feel to have achieved this goal?

Pause

Low Carbohydrate Diet

Now, I want you to join me on a fun exercise where we will play a little game using your imagination.

Picture a full platter of freshly cut, delicious, and colourful fruits and vegetables.

Pause

As you take a closer look at the platter, you notice how fresh and delicious the fruits look, and as you begin to smell the fragrance of your favourite fruits, you start to salivate.

Pause

You pick up your favourite fruit, and you take a crunchy bite, and you immediately feel the delicious flavours ooze into your mouth, and you can sense your taste buds dancing with joy.

Longer Pause

There was a time when you had overlooked these beautiful fruits and vegetables, but today you realise the importance and goodness of it. And you have now consciously made the decision to switch to a low carb diet which is another wise decision toward a healthier and active lifestyle.

Pause

You are now fully aware of all the health benefits that come with eating nutritious foods. You understand that it not only helps you lose weight but it also significantly helps you stay mentally alert.

Nutritious food helps you get through the day effortlessly.

A nutritious diet consists of lean proteins, fruits and vegetables, and whole grains, and these foods feed your body with minerals and vitamins which are essential for a healthy body and mind.

It is important to maintain a healthy balance of carbohydrates and proteins as they are an excellent source of energy.

Vegetables and fruits are a great source of fiber which keep your stomach full for longer periods of time.

The darker the veggies, the more nutrients they contain.

With this well balanced diet, you will have beautiful, glowing skin, and an attractive body. You will be completely transformed, and you are looking forward excitedly to living a life full of confidence, with an active slim body, and clear, glowing skin.

And this is all going to be possible only because you have made these great decisions today.

Longer Pause

Today you are taking your first steps into the universe of healthy and nutritious foods, of eating mindfully, and taking time to nurture your mind and body.

This is going to help you feel fitter, lighter and you will be brimming with confidence.

Pause

Now I want you to imagine all this healthy food entering your body, and nurturing your body with all the essential nutrients.

You now know that a low carb diet provides your body with small doses of insulin which gets stored in the body as good fat, and is a great source of energy.

A low carb diet leaves no room for fat backlog, and it in fact helps you lose weight too.

Now, use your imagination and picture the insides of your stomach, and take a close look at how light and healthy your stomach feels. How happy and clean your intestines feel after you have switched to a healthy and nutritious diet.

Pause

You are now very aware of the advantages of switching to a low carb diet.

A few of these benefits include weight loss, reduction in the fat stored in your body, and high levels of energy.

And with this knowledge, you can now tick off the low calorie, non-starchy, and protein-rich diet as a success.

Pause

From this moment on, you will be eating a healthier, nutritious diet in small portions to keep your stomach and yourself happy which will help you steadily move toward your weight loss goal.

Pause

You are now more mindful of your diet because of which you have embraced protein-rich, low-carb foods, and colourful and fresh fruits and vegetables.

You now consciously take smaller portions of food spread across six meals per day, and you drink at least eight glasses of water.

You are focussed about eating right and exercising each and every day as that brings you closer to your larger goal of weight loss.

Pause

Now, I would like you to pay close attention to the suggestions I am about share with you, and repeat it in your mind

I eat healthy foods (4 seconds pauses)

I eat smaller portions (4 seconds pauses)

I exercise regularly (4 seconds pauses)

I am conscious of my eating habits (4 seconds pauses)

I eat mindfully (4 seconds pauses)

I exercise regularly (4 seconds pauses)

Pause

Self-Hypnosis

Now, observe as you begin to feel a soothing sensation take over your entire body, all the way from your toes to the top of your head.

Imagine your body releasing all tension and worries as it gently falls into a deep state of relaxation and peacefulness.

Pause

Visualise this peaceful, relaxing feeling as it gently moves upward from your toes, to your ankles, lower legs, to your hips, lower arms, elbows, your upper arms and shoulder through to your neck, back, face and all the way up to your head.

Allow your entire body to sink deeply into the surface where you are sitting or lying down, and gently visualise yourself slowly walking down toward the ocean.

Imagine yourself walking down through a blissfully green tropical forest with tall green trees all around providing you with the perfect shade from the sun.

And as you keep walking, you can softly hear the sound of the waves crashing, you can faintly smell the ocean, and you can feel a gentle breeze brush against you which gives you a very pleasant feeling.

Pause

You now begin to see the beautiful turquoise waters of the ocean as you slowly come to the end of the walking path and onto the warm sandy shores of the ocean.

You take off your shoes and sink your feet into the soft white sand. The sand is nice and warm and makes you feel calm and relaxed.

Notice how long and far the beach stretches to your left and to your right, and notice the sun shine glistening off the water far into the horizon.

Observe the water slowly swelling up and forming waves as they come crashing against the coastline one after the other in a very systematic, and rhythmic pattern.

Pause

Now imagine yourself slowly walking toward the water, your feet sinking into the soft warm sand, and as you keep walking, you begin to feel the heat of the sun, and you start feeling very hot.

As you get closer to the water, you feel the ocean mist gently kiss your skin, and as you keep walking, the texture of the sand is now wet and firm.

You feel a wave wash over your feet as it continues to race up the banks, crash and recede back into the sea.

Pause

As you step forward, you feel more and more waves splash against your feet. The coolness of the water gives you a much needed relief from the heat.

The water is clear, clean and pleasant, and you can easily see the surface as you keep walking further into the ocean.

You can continue to walk further if you wish or take a leisurely swim.

You feel a real sense of joy as you spend more time floating in the water, and you begin to feel deeply relaxed.

You feel extremely calm and refreshed.

Now you gently get back on your feet and start walking back out of the water.

And as you gently stroll along the beach, you feel a sense of relief. All your stress and worries have all been washed away.

As you continue to walk back, you notice a comfortable lounge chair and towel waiting for you.

You lay down the towel on the chair, and gently lie down enjoying the sun, the breeze and the waves.

You lay there and enjoy the stillness for a few more moments.

Now, whenever you're ready gently bring your focus back from this visual vacation.

You begin to slowly bring your focus back to your body, noticing the sensation at the sole of your feet, and you feel the weight of your body against the bed.

You feel completely recharged and rejuvenated, ready to return to your day with a refreshed mind.

Now gently open your eyes, and stretch your arms and legs as you become fully alert of your surroundings.

And remember you can practise this visual relaxation anywhere, at any time of the day. And with each practise you will become more and more skilled at effectively refreshing your mind and body.

Protective Sleep

I would like to take a moment here to talk to you about the difficulties you have been facing of late in trying to get some deep sleep. One of the reasons owing to which this tends to happen is when the subconsious part of your mind assumes the role of a protector. That is to say that while a part of your mind may be trying to get you to sleep peacefully, there is a part that is on high alert, as if on the lookout for any threats or events that may possibly occur at night.

Pause

However, this was not always the case, for in the past you have had someone to keep an eye out for you as you slept peacefully through the night. Be it your parents who may have checked in on you to ensure you slept well and were secure, or a partner who slept beside you, or even a pet guarding you or to alert you should the need arise.

Pause

And of late, for one reason or another, somewhere deep in your mind you feel as if the protection you had in the past is no longer there, so you must watch out for yourself on your own.

And for this reason the unconscious part of your mind feels the need to avoid sleeping in order to keep you secure.

Let me take a moment here to assure you that there is no longer any need for the unconscious part of your mind to assume such responsibility and stay on high alert through the night. I say this because there is someone else who assumes the responsibility of keeping you safe and guarding you through the night as you sleep -- watching over you, and that is your guide to protect you. It could be an angel or the one you truly believe will protect and watch over you.

Pause

Your guide is someone who has immense love for you. This guide could even be one of those people who were dear to you, who protected you through the night in the past, but may have since passed on. Though they may not be here with you physically, they are watching over you and ensuring you stay safe at all times, especially during the night.

Pause

And though you may, by now have a fair idea of who this might be, it isn't important, because what matters is that there is someone guarding and protecting you at all times, and this someone loves you very, very much. You may not see them, you may not even feel their physical presence at all -- but they are always there, like a warm, cosy cocoon of safety that resides within your heart as you sleep.

I will now be helping you understand and be able to feel the presence of your guide

as they watch over you and protect you.

Start by relaxing your body slowly and steadily, all the way starting from your toes and ankles. Follow the rhythm of your breath -- breathing in relaxation and breathing out any muscle tension you may feel throughout your body. Let this relaxation move up from your ankles, filling up your shins and calves, as it slowly makes its way to settle into your thighs making you feel twice as relaxed and at ease before moving further up and relaxing your waist and lower back. Feel this heavy relaxation settling into your stomach and back, making its way into your chest and shoulders, all the way through your arms and into your fingertips. Breathe in more relaxation and let go of any muscle tension in your neck, jaw, cheeks, and forehead, all the way to the top of your head. that's right, your entire body is full to the brim with this heavy and peaceful relaxation.

Pause

And now that every part of your body is deeply relaxed, visualise yourself standing at the very top of a grand, beautiful staircase that leads you to a place very special to you, making you feel calmer, more relaxed, and sleepier. As you take a good look at this staircase, you notice how safe and relaxing it feels.

You notice the number of steps on this staircase and you can even notice how relaxing it is to know that it leads to a place that is so special to you.

Pause

Slowly begin descending these stairs, counting yourself down with each step. With each step you take, you find a heavy relaxation sinking into you, making you feel calm and safe. The further down you go, the more relaxed you become. Slowly and steadily everything around you begins to feel a little distant and vague, as if everything was slowly fading away with each step taking you deeper and deeper into relaxation. By the time you reach the very bottom of this staircase, you are so deeply relaxed that the world around you would have gradually faded away, leaving you in your special place to relax. This special place could be a pristine sandy beach or a beautiful garden, maybe you find yourself sitting and enjoying the sunset. Whatever and wherever it may be, allow your mind to simply drift away and wander in this special place.

Pause

As your mind continues to wander, you begin to drift with it, into a calming and relaxing feeling. You feel comfortable, as if wrapped in a warm blanket. Drifting further and further, deeper and deeper, feeling more and more relaxed.

By now you are so deeply and heavily relaxed that any thoughts or ideas or images cropping up in your mind barely make it into your conscious awareness, they just float away, leaving you more and more relaxed.

Pause

Maybe at this point you are so relaxed that even my voice seems to have become softer as if coming from quite far away. And in a few short moments, you will find yourself drifting into a short peaceful sleep. And while you may sleep for a short while, you will be able to return to this relaxing hypnotic rest when I speak your name. The moment you hear my voice calling out your name, you will return to this peaceful hypnotic rest, but for now you are slowly drifting into a very calming and tranquil sleep.

As you continue to enjoy this peaceful sleep, you will dream about all the memories that make you feel warm and cosy, almost childlike, filling up your heart with so much love, more than it can carry, so the love fills up your entire body, every nook and corner, making you feel twice as deeply relaxed and brimming with joy.

As this feeling continues to grow within you, you find yourself faced with the realization that you are not alone in feeling all this love and joy and warmth. That out there in a parallel plane of life, there is someone who shares this feeling with you, who loves you just as deeply as you love them. And you soon realise that they are watching over you in a very special way, making you feel so safe and deeply relaxed that you find yourself drifting further and further, deeper and deeper into a state where sleep comes to you with so much ease.

Pause

Soak it all in. Take a few moments here to take in all the love, joy, and tranquility that this moment and this realization brings with itself. Enjoy every bit of this feeling.

That's right.

Pause

And now, from this very moment, you are capable of naturally and easily drifting into a peaceful and relaxing deep sleep whenever you so desire. You are able to find yourself settling into a relaxing hypnotic rest whenever you feel you are ready to sleep. And from there you will drift into your special place, just like right now, and in that special place you will find yourself feeling every bit of the love and protection from your guide. And as your guide will protect you through the night, you will find yourself drifting into deep sleep with ease.

Pause

You are capable of sleeping for as long as you desire, and should you awaken in the middle of the night, you will easily and naturally return to deep sleep by simply tapping into this relaxing state of hypnotic rest.

Relaxing Sleep

Every time you want to fall asleep, you can simply begin by relaxing your physical body in the same way as you have done today. Begin by closing your eyes, taking a deep breath and then scanning and relaxing each part of your body from your toes all the way up to the top of your head.

Pause

You will feel a heavy sense of relaxation sinking into you as you scan your toes and ankles, your shins and calves, going up to your knees and thighs, gently relaxing your hips, your waist, and your lower back as you scan your way up to your stomach and your back, moving to your chest, relaxing your heart, feeling the relaxation building up in your arms and fingers, and as you scan your neck, jaw, eyes, forehead and head you feel absolutely relaxed inside-out.

Pause

Once this heavy sense of relaxation has settled into every part of you, you can picture yourself standing at the very top of a majestic staircase. This staircase leads you to a place that is very special to you. A place where you feel completely safe, at ease, and very very sleepy.

Begin to count yourself down as you begin descending this staircase slowly and steadily. The further down you go, the more relaxed and sleepy you feel. And as you descend through this majestic staircase you will begin to feel the world around you fading away the more relaxed you feel, and this makes you even sleepier. At the bottom of the staircase you find yourself in a very special and safe place -- it could be a garden, a beach, a meadow, or even the mountains, where you can sit or lie down comfortably as you watch the sunset. So let your mind drift and let it take you to this special place. Let go. As you begin to let yourself go, you find yourself surrounded by a warm cosy mist.

Pause

And just like this mist, let yourself drift to where your mind takes you. There is no need to think, just sit back and observe from a distance. Notice the sights and images that crop up through your subconscious mind as they gently float and drift along with you. Softly and slowly, drifting and floating, floating and drifting, slowly and slowly.

As your mind continues to float slowly along with this comfortable and warm mist, you feel deeply relaxed and safe. You feel joy filling you up from within as you continue moving along and drifting with the mist, freely floating. You feel more and more deeply relaxed, sleepier and sleepier than ever before.

Pause

A few moments from now, you will find yourself gently settling into a short sleep. And for now, continue to picture and enjoy this cosy mist settling into this special place around you. Little by little the entire landscape begins to fill up with this mist, so soft and comfortable. The mist starts to become thicker and thicker, making you feel more and more comfortable and deeply relaxed. The thicker the mist becomes, the more at ease and sleepier you become.

Pause

So, let this mist grow thicker and wrap your special place with lots of warmth and comfort. The more you do so, the more you notice how various thoughts, images, feelings, and memories begin to drift in and out of your awareness. You are so deeply relaxed and sleepy that they pass you by without entering your awareness as you continue to focus on the sound of my voice. The more you pay attention to the sound of my voice, the dimmer these thoughts and memories become. They seem to fade away every now and then and you become more and more relaxed.

Pause

You are now completely wrapped up in this warm, cosy, and soft mist that makes you feel so comfortable and relaxed in every nook and corner of your body. All of the thoughts, feelings, and memories have faded so much they almost seem vague. Even my voice by now seems to have become more distant as if it were fading away too, leaving you more and more relaxed and at ease.

Any thoughts that do make their way into your awareness seem to fade away quickly, leaving you more relaxed. And with each passing moment, it begins to get more and more misty, all the thoughts and feelings and ideas fade in and out of your awareness, becoming more and more vague with each passing moment, as the mist continues to thicken, my voice becomes fainter as if coming from further and further away.

Pause

It may seem like my voice is becoming more and more distant, fainter and fainter with each passing moment as you continue to drift further and further. Floating away in the mist feeling more and more relaxed, comfortable, and sleepier. You find yourself drifting further down within yourself, becoming sleepier and deeply relaxed, down into a naturally sound sleep.

Pause

You will only sleep for a short while, and then soon after you will be able to hear my voice calling your name. When you do notice my voice calling your name, you will find yourself slowly coming out of this short sleep and returning to a peaceful state of hypnotic rest.

Pause

You are now drifting deeper and deeper. Everything around you is becoming more and more vague as you drift away into a comfortable sleep.

Pause

Great, from now on you are able to gently float into a restful sleep whenever you desire to do so. You will be able to drift into a peaceful hypnotic rest as you get ready to go to sleep, following which you will find yourself in your special place, being surrounded with a warm and cosy mist, with all your thoughts and feelings fading away slowly as you fall asleep. You can sleep for as long as you desire and wake up easily, feeling refreshed.

Be Healthy

When you are trying to achieve your ideal weight goal, you are not only looking at eating the right food, but you also looking at including at least 30 minutes of exercise into your daily routine.

And as you begin to enjoy this process, it becomes easier for you to achieve your goal.

Staying focussed and motivated about achieving your weight loss goal is very essential in achieving the end result.

Pause

Now picture yourself in the future where you are confident, attractive and healthy, and when you look at your future self, you will feel proud of all the efforts you took to make this possible.

Your focus and motivation to eat right, exercise regularly, and staying positive during the difficult periods has helped you achieve your goal.

And you realise how you continued to grow in confidence with every step you took toward a healthier and happier lifestyle.

Now, think of all the benefits that come with weight loss, and notice how you feel, and note what kind of activities you are looking forward to.

Longer Pause

And as you make a mental note of all the activities you would enjoy, I want you to listen to my words carefully, and repeat it to yourself in your mind.

I am slimmer (10 seconds pause)

I am releasing extra weight (10 seconds pause)

I am confident (10 seconds pause)

I love myself (10 seconds pause)

I am fit (10 seconds pause)

I am excited to lose weight (10 seconds pause)

I am motivated to lose weight (10 seconds pause)

I exercise regularly (10 seconds pause)

I eat well and in smaller portions (10 seconds pause)

Be More Active

Continue to keep a gentle focus on your breath, and let yourself breathe naturally as you drift deeper and deeper into a relaxed state of mind.

And pay close attention to every word I say while keeping an open mind because each and every word is intended with a greater purpose to help you achieve your larger goal.

You are a loveable individual, and from this moment on, you will be confident, and you will be in complete control of your thoughts and actions.

You will be mindful of your eating habits, and you will consciously choose healthier and nutritious food options.

Longer Pause

You will immediately recognize your emotional triggers such as when you are bored or feeling down, and you will be mindful to navigate these challenges in a relaxed and confident manner.

You will engage yourself in physical activities such as walking, running and exercising daily.

You will spend time connecting with your friends, family and loved ones.

You will use constructive methods to unwind or divert your attention by watching light hearted content when you need a laugh, or you will spend time reading a book.

Pause

You will take control of what you eat, and you will reach the ideal goal weight by choosing healthy and nutritious foods.

You will also spend 30 to 40 minutes exercising every day, and this is going to help you lose weight and reach your goal faster.

Pause

You can split your exercise routine into two parts. You could do 15 minutes in the morning, and 30 minutes later in the day or vice versa.

With each passing day, you will slowly feel physically and mentally more upbeat which will give you the energy and motivation to exercise more.

You will look and feel confident, toned, attractive and happy.

And as you progress, you will continue to constantly lose weight and tone up in a healthy manner.

Maintenance Insomnia Relaxation

When we go to sleep at night, we do not really follow a process of falling asleep -- we just do., because we just know how to. Sleep is natural and simple, and a good night's sleep is capable of making us feel refreshed, energized, and rejuvenated and ready to start our day and get things done as we go about our daily living.

However, for some people, this simple and natural course of sleep may get interrupted as they may awaken due to unwelcome and unwanted thoughts cluttering their mind, making it difficult for them to rest and fall asleep or stay asleep. The longer these thoughts linger, the harder it becomes for them to fall asleep.

Pause

The Law of Reversed Effect in Hypnosis, or as we often call it Coue's Law, suggests a reason for this, and that reason being, the more we try to remember or the more we try to do something, the more difficult it becomes for us to remember or do it. So, the more one tries to escape the intrusive thoughts and fall asleep, the more difficult it becomes to do so.

Pause

You may have noticed it too. Perhaps while trying to remember someone's name or even a word to describe something -- no matter how much you try you just can't seem to remember what it was until much later when you are not actively trying to remember it, and it suddenly dawns on you almost out of nowhere!

Pause

The solution? To stop trying and let go. The only way to beat the Law of Reversed Effect is to stop fighting it. This is exactly how we are going to win against the problem you have been experiencing lately -- of awakening in the middle of your sleep, and then trying and trying very hard to go back to sleep.

The solution to this problem, as mentioned before, is to simply stop trying and to stop putting in any effort to fall back asleep. The moment you let go, you will fall asleep just like that. As if it was always that easy and natural.

Pause

Whenever you find yourself awakening in the middle of your sleep, you will simply put away the thought of sleeping from your mind. You can instead think about anything and everything else -- planning for the next day, the things you need to get done, prioritising and deciding what could be done first and what could be done last, or maybe even solving a riddle someone asked you a while ago, or rehearse some activity you were planning to do. You can think of just about anything. You may even get up from your bed and do something else -- perhaps a task you had long been putting off for later. But the one thing you absolutely cannot do is to think of falling asleep.

And soon when the next day arrives, you will wake up to find yourself having slept and slept well. That sleep came so easily and naturally to you, without any effort. You will find yourself surprised at how easy it was, one moment you were planning your activities for the next day, and the next moment you wake up fully relaxed and energised to begin your day after a restful sleep full of sweet dreams that gently lulled you back to sleep.

Pause

From this moment on, the most efficient tool you have is that of letting go. Let go of the perry or the need to fall back asleep any time you find yourself awake at odd hours. Simply use that time to plan and rehearse and reflect on the things that are on priority and need to be done. Complete a few chores if you have to -- anything but trying to go back to sleep. And you will find yourself drifting into a state of relaxing deep sleep without you even noticing it. And when you wake up refreshed the next day, you won't even be able to pinpoint when or how you went back to sleep, but you did, and now you are well rested and free from the worries that no longer hold importance in your life.

Pause

You are now able to remind yourself to remember that you must forget about trying to or even thinking about sleep, for it is something very natural and easy and simple, and it will come to you naturally and easily. Eventually, you will find yourself so adept at remembering to forget about sleep that you will most naturally begin sleeping peacefully every single night without awakening in between even once, only waking up at the regular time the next day feeling fresh and full of motivation to get things done and have a great day -- all because now you are in the habit of getting a good night's sleep every night.

Pause

You can so easily now remember to forget to remember to sleep, and when you forget to remember to go back to sleep, you will find yourself resting through the night in a good night's sleep every time and only awakening the next morning at the scheduled time to get started with your day. Just remember this and you will be fine.

Inner Strength and Power

If you continue listening to every word I say with utmost concentration and enthusiasm, you go into an even intense, deeper, and relaxed state of mind and body. Your imagination is carrying you to a lovely green meadow in your mind, a meadow full of fresh green plants, trees, and hills. The beautiful green meadow is surrounded by lots of flowers in different colors like blue, yellow, red, white, and the ones that are your favorite. Imagine yourself walking through the meadow in a fresh and pure atmosphere.

Longer Pause
You are now looking up at the sky and you see a stretch of the bluish bright skyline with a hint of rays from the sun. It is a beautiful, warm day with a slight breeze that is making you feel like you are in a movie. As you keep moving ahead, appreciating nature's charm, you see a path that leads to a grand beach. You continue walking towards the beach feeling calm and blessed.

Longer Pause

Once you reach the beach you take off your shoes and feel the warm, fine-grained, white sand on the skin of your body. As you start wandering on the sand for few minutes, you find a very relaxing lounge with a bonfire. You get excited and sit by the fire. You take a glance around and you notice there is only you as far as your eyes can see. Gradually you feel a wave of tenderness and realize that even you are sitting beside a bonfire you have a very heavy coat on your body.

You realize that even though you have had it for a while now you have noticed it just now. You reach through the pocket of your coat and you find a small piece of paper in there. The paper has a name written on it of someone that you are not very fond of and someone who stresses you out most of the time. The reason for the stress caused by the person is very clearly mentioned on the paper. You look carefully at everything that the paper reads (get an ideomotor response). After having a glance thoroughly, you crumble the paper and throw it into the fire. You watch the paper slowly turning into ashes, you see the black smoke rise up and disappear in the air.

This is making you happy. You search your pocket one more time and once again you find a piece of paper in it. The paper has a name on it of someone you know and someone who stresses you out most of the time. The paper also points the reasons why this person is the reason for your stress.

Look carefully at everything that it mentions. After reading it you crumble the paper and throw it into the fire. You watch the paper burning and the smoke from it disappearing in the air.

Longer Pause

This makes you happy but a little annoyed as well this time. Once again you decide to dig into your pocket and this time as well you find one. You wonder what is going on. When you pull your hand out from the pocket, you bring a handful of little chits with more names written on it of all the people and circumstances that have troubled, outraged, or have hurt you at some or other point in life. You get angry and throw all the papers in the fire and as each paper turns into ashes, it makes you lighter and happier. You lift your left index paper when all the papers have been turned to ashes.

You feel light as if you're whole body has been released from agony. You feel free as a bird. You then decide to throw your coat into the bonfire as well. You want to experience freedom and don't want any kind of heaviness weighing you down in any way. You close your eyes, take a deep breath in and out and feel calm.

Pause

You now begin to hear a vague sound, something like a waterfall that is far away. You start walking towards the sound, the sound gets clearer when you move towards it, and you then find that it is certainly a grand waterfall with a huge pond of fresh blue water, nothing like you have seen before.

The sound of the water from the fall makes you happy and homely. The place where you can connect yourself with no guilt and opinion, a place that gives you inner strength and peace. Here, if you wish to swim into the water and have pleasure, then you just have to live up to your index finger. Now, you can fearlessly move forward and dive in (give them a few minutes)

Just stand under the fall and try to grab all the natural wonders that surround you. As the fresh, clean and cold water touches your body and flows from above your body to your toes, you feel it is cleansing and taking you away from the insecurities, doubts, and fears contained inside you, especially about your weight.

Pause

You let the water carry away all the negativity that is stored inside you and that goes everywhere you go- from your body far away with the water, let everything go. (Get an ideomotor response when this feels complete to them)

The strength inside your mind and body is rising and glowing. Space that was filled with negativity and bad thoughts is now replaced by happy thoughts and positive energy. You are in love with yourself all over again, you bond much stronger with your inner self this time. Let this feeling sink in and thank the waterfall for providing everything you need to stay happy, calm, and joyful.

(Have them stay with the image as long as you feel it's appropriate, repeating some of these positive words)

It's now the time to remember and thank all the amazing places that you strolled in your mind. Thank the beach, the waterfall, the beautiful meadow for teaching you new things and for bringing positivity and hope in your life.

Suggestions

"Now's the time to make some important conclusions that will adversely affect you."
(Pause)

"With more energy and good vibes, your body is becoming tougher and healthier than it used to be before" (or however they want their body to look and feel)
"You feel great and your body looks perfect"
"Now you only want a healthy diet, you hate sitting idle and you love exercising daily"
"You are gaining more and more confidence each passing day"
"You are happy with everything in all aspects of your existence. You might not realize this at the minute but its completely fine, the more you try, the more suggestions will come your way and will transform you into an amazing way"

Connect with Your Special Place

This is a meditation that is making you feel good about yourself, is going to calm and relax your body and mind, and is going to help you imagine a special place for yourself. This is a place where you are going to feel special and at peace. Therefore, now allow yourself to go into this special place.

It is going to be either indoors or outdoors and is a very special and secure place. I would love you to continue imagining this amazing place. You must become aware of how it feels to be there...

Sense the smell captures the beauty and notices everything that you see.

Longer Pause

Now find a place where you comfortably sit. As you sit, try to feel the place beneath you. Now I am wondering if you could make this place even better and charming. You will feel empowered even just by spending time over there.

Longer Pause

When you sit in your special place you will find
yourself at your ideal goal weight.

Longer Pause

Have a strong belief in yourself

You are a very confident woman and you believe in yourself, you are aware of your capabilities, and trust your choices. You have certain qualities that are appreciated by all. Try and recall them as I take a few minutes off.

Longer Pause of 20 seconds

People appreciate you for who you are as a human being and like you for the qualities that you possess.

Now I wonder if you remember your top 5 best qualities. They could either be simple, usual, or unusual, it depends. Just get the knowledge of these.

Longer Pause

What are some of the other reasons that make people like you or drawn to you?

Longer Pause
You are a strong independent woman and a very confident person. As you recall these

superb traits that you possess, you feel more confident, strong, and superior.

Confidence in your abilities
You know that you are capable of achieving anything and everything that you put your mind to or get on the path of achieving it.

You are well aware that you can finish any task perfectly and on time with the right execution. And I even wonder if you have a goal that you want to achieve in your mind.

Pause

As soon as you think about the goal that you have in your mind, I would love you to imagine wondering about it and thinking about how to achieve it. You have done a lot, shed off your blood and tears to achieve this goal, now you only have to take the right actions so that it could be achieved with precision and with perfection.

When you recall your preparation it will automatically boost your confidence because you have worked hard and are well prepared for it. And according to the record, if a person prepares well and in advance, is worthy enough to execute it in an even better way and finish it with perfection. Be it any goal, doesn't matter.

The goal could either be eating healthy or exercising regularly. You even know that if you prepare yourself mentally, you can achieve the goal easily and with perfection. You just have to prepare for it with dedication. For example, if the goal is going for jogging or hitting workout sessions, you can go for it by putting on an alarm, keeping your socks and shoes out, and keeping your sportswear out.

As you prepare you to feel confident enough that you are going to achieve this goal. And as you are out to achieve the goal, you will accomplish it. This will boost your confidence to another level and make you into a truly confident woman.

Pause

And from now onwards, you are this super confident, strong-headed, and focused woman. Every time you prepare for achieving something, you are confident enough that you will perform with great dedication and will be at your best.

Longer Pause

You trust and respect yourself which is of utmost importance, people respect you. And as you are thinking about this I wonder if you can press your index finger against your thumb and say the word- confidence with confidence. And if you will notice that if you press them hard against each other your confidence doubles and if you press it harder it triples up.

Pause

This means that anytime you need to feel confident enough in a certain situation or boost it harder, you simply have to press your index finger against your thumb and you will be filled with immense positivity, confidence, and enthusiasm to tackle any situation better.

This makes you confident enough to achieve your goals, confident enough to talk to people around you with assertiveness. With this, you set boundaries that are easy for you, and this, in turn, raises your self-esteem and self-confidence.

Affirmations

1. You enjoy eating raw, fresh fruits and vegetables every single day and savor their flavors. (Pause for 10 seconds)
2. You are motivated to hit the gym and workout regularly(same as above)
3. Your positivity is increasing with your growth and you are becoming more positive as you progress. (same as above)
4. You are now more focused on your daily actions and daily goals(same as above)
5. You can visualize yourself at your ideal weight and all the outcomes and benefit that come with that(same as above)
6. You stay attentive and focused on this weight loss journey that you are going on(same as above)
7. You love the aroma and the taste of this raw healthy food (same as above)
8. You enjoy the taste, flavors, and colors of fresh vegetables and fruits. (same as above)
9. You have started including lean protein and dairy products like skimmed milk in your diet. (same as above)
10. You have even started to enjoy the taste of salads(same as above)
11. You are becoming thinner and thinner day by day(same as above)

12. Your waist is getting smaller, slimmer, and in shape(same as above)
13. You are getting leaner and stronger with each passing because of the hard work that you put in(same as above)
14. You are gaining muscles and shedding off the extra mass that you hate on your body(same as above)
15. You feel strong and confident every single day and this motivates you to do better than ever(same as above)
16. By trusting your body and mind it is getting easier and easier for you to trust yourself. (same as before)
17. Your health is getting better and is improving every day. (same as above)
18. You now can make smaller changes for the highest good. (same as above)
19. You have become more confident, patient and have started to believe in yourself a lot more(same as above)
20. You trust yourself that you are on the right journey, the journey that will take you towards your goal(same as above)
21. You easily let go of the past mistakes that you committed(same as above)
22. You are against emotional eating and you can easily say no to it. (same as before)
23. Weight loss is becoming easier and better for you day by day(same as before)
24. You feel positive, energetic, and enthusiastic after waking up(same as before)

25. Your future is in your hands and you are solely responsible for it(same as before)
26. You have gained more belief in your strengths and capabilities(same as before)
27. You are capable of losing the extra mass off your body(same as above)
28. You love yourself more than before and you take care of your mind and body with the most dedication. (same as before)
29. You are contained with love and brimming with self-care (same as above)
30. You intake foods that are healthy and rich in nutrients(same as above)
31. Your confidence is boosting every day(same as above)
32. You are brimming with confidence(same as above)
33. You trust and believe yourself(same as above)
34. Your self-love and care is increasing every day(same as above)
35. You are now more focused on this journey of weight loss(same as above)
36. You are getting fitter and in shape(same as above)
37. The right choices that you make are sailing you through this journey of weight loss(7 seconds pause)
38. Everyone around you is supporting and applauding you for your sheer dedication and hard work(7 seconds pause)

39. You constantly imagine yourself at your ideal weight, the goal weight that you have in your mind(7 seconds pause)
40. You are mindful of eating healthy and fresh(7 seconds pause)
41. You easily deny the offer of unhealthy food(7 seconds pause)
42. Your body is in sync with your mind and together these two is doing wonders(7 seconds pause)
43. You eat only when you are physically starving(7 seconds pause)
44. You are excited that you will achieve your goal weight and even more excited about how you will maintain it. (7 seconds pause)
45. You are permanently and easily losing weight(7 seconds pause)
46. You are in love with your body and enjoy yourself in this journey that will help you earn your desired body through the hard work that you put in(7 seconds pause)
47. You are shedding off extra mass(7 seconds pause)
48. You are satisfying your appetite by taking the right food in the right proportion(7 seconds pause)
49. You work out daily (7 seconds pause)
50. You are well aware of your eating schedule(7 seconds pause)
51. You like to watch content on weight loss and healthy food every day, it motivates you to do better and better(7 seconds pause)

52. You are excited to work on your mind and body consistently and with dedication(7 seconds pause)
53. Your body and its every cell is getting healed(7 seconds pause)
54. Every day you offer gratitude and wake up with the feeling of gratefulness(7 seconds pause)
55. You trust the cycle of life and even more trust yourself(7 seconds pause)
56. You are well aware of the capabilities of your body and mind(7 seconds pause)
57. Your love for yourself is unconditional and pure(7 seconds pause)
58. You are gracious and compassionate towards yourself(7 seconds pause)
59. You eat healthily and enjoy every mouthful(7 seconds pause)
60. You chew every bite many times and enjoy the flavors (7 seconds pause)
61. You are capable of doing wonders(7 seconds pause)
62. You deserve all the love and care that life has to offer(7 seconds pause)
63. You work out regularly and take care of your health(7 seconds pause)
64. You are filled with confidence and courage(7 seconds pause)
65. You forgive yourself for all the past mistakes(7 seconds pause)
66. You like to stay in the present and are more mindful(7 seconds pause)

67. You know when and how to say no to emotional eating(7 seconds pause)
68. You are conscious about what and how you eat(7 seconds pause)
69. You have daily goals of exercises and eating right in proportion(7 seconds pause)
70. You stuff yourself only when you are actually hungry(7 seconds pause)
71. You enjoy this journey of weight loss(7 seconds pause)
72. You enjoy each day of this journey(7 seconds pause)
73. The result starts to appear soon in front of you(7 seconds pause)
74. Every day you are becoming more confident and courageous(7 seconds pause)
75. You are getting fitter and more desirable with every passing day(7 seconds pause)
76. You are enjoying your life even better by eating healthy and in the right amount(7 seconds pause)
77. You love your body with all your heart(7 seconds pause)
78. You eat healthy food which is rich in nutrients and is of great value(7 seconds pause)
79. You eat fruits and vegetables in different colors (7 seconds pause)
80. You can easily identify the difference between mental and physical hunger(7 seconds pause)

81. You make the right choices about your diet(7 seconds pause)
82. You enjoy each day(7 seconds pause)
83. You are motivated enough to achieve your target(7 seconds pause)
84. You work out daily at least for 30 minutes(7 seconds pause)
85. You get amazed by the progress you see in the mirror(7 seconds pause)
86. You often listen to the saved recordings(7 seconds pause)
87. You have high self-confidence(7 seconds pause)
88. You are worthy(7 seconds pause)
89. You are desirable(7 seconds pause)
90. You are fitter than ever(7 seconds pause)
91. Most often you are in good mood(7 seconds pause)
92. You are happy and full of positivity(7 seconds pause)
93. You allow positive energy to surround you every day(7 seconds pause)
94. You choose to look at the glass half or full daily(7 seconds pause)
95. You are thankful for everything(7 seconds pause)
96. As soon as you get on the bed you fall asleep(7 seconds pause)
97. As soon as you press your index finger against your thumb you feel calm and relaxed(7 seconds pause)

98. You are becoming leaner and fitter(7 seconds pause)
99. You look beautiful and happy(7 seconds pause)
100. You take care of your body beautifully(7 seconds pause)
101. You take immense care of your body (7 seconds pause)
102. You appreciate eating raw fresh fruits every day and love to savor their flavors (Pause for another 10 seconds)
103. You want to exercise every day. (same as above)
104. You are giving positive rays as you progressing. (same as above)
105. You are now more focused on your goals and daily actions(same as above)
106. You can now easily visualize yourself at the weight you always desired, the weight which comes with a lot of benefits(same as above)
107. Stay focused on this journey of fat loss(same as above)
108. You are now enjoying the taste of raw healthy meals(same as above)
109. You are enjoying the taste of fresh fruits and vegetables(same as above)
110. You are now including lean protein and skimmed milk in your diet(same as above)
111. You are enjoying the flavors of salad(same as above)
112. You are becoming leaner and leaner day by day. (same as above)

113. Your waist is becoming slimmer with each passing day. (same as above)
114. You are getting tougher and stronger every day. (same as above)
115. You are losing weight and gaining power(same as above)
116. You feel healthier than before(same as above)
117. By trusting your body you are now able to trust yourself easily(same as above)
118. Your health is upgrading every single day(same as above)
119. You now can bring in small changes for the highest goods. (same as above)
120. You have become patient and you tend to believe more in yourself(same as above)
121. You believe that you are on the right path(same as above)
122. Now you can easily let go of the past(same as above)
123. You are against emotional easting(same as above)
124. Weight loss has become easier for you(same as above)
125. You feel new energy after waking up(same as above)
126. You are the creator of your future(same as above)
127. You are gaining confidence in your fortes and capabilities(same as above)
128. You have the power of becoming an ideal person(same as above(

129. You are in love with yourself even more than before and this is making you take care of your mind and body(same as before)

130. You are blossoming with love and care(same as before)

131. You consume high food rich in nutrients(same as before)

132. Your confidence is on another level these days(same as before)

133. You are confident and believe in yourself(same as above)

134. You trust your worth(same as above)

135. Your self-love and care is accelerating(same as above)

136. You are more focusing on your goal, the goal to reach your ideal weight(same as above)

137. You are getting slimmer and leaner(7 seconds pause)

138. Your ability to make the right decisions is helping you to move further in this game of weight loss (7 seconds pause)

139. Every soul surrounding you is applauding you(7 seconds pause)

140. You constantly imagine yourself being at your goal(7 seconds pause)

141. You are mindful of eating raw and fresh(7 seconds pause)

142. Now you easily deny unhealthy eating habits(7 seconds pause)

143. Your body is syncing with your mind(7 seconds pause)

144. You eat only when you are hungry(7 seconds pause)

145. You are excited by the fact that you will achieve your ideal weight(7 seconds pause)

146. You are getting rid of the fat permanently(7 seconds pause)

147. You love this journey of moving towards your ideal weight, the journey which is leading you to achieve your desired body(7 seconds pause)

148. You are getting rid of the masses (7 seconds pause)

149. You are eating the right amount of food in the right proportion that is required for losing weight(7 seconds pause)

150. You exercise every day(7 seconds pause)

151. You are mindful of your eating patterns(7 seconds pause)

152. You gain knowledge about weight loss and healthy food every day (7 seconds pause)

153. You are enthusiastic about working towards the goal that you have(7 seconds pause)

154. Your cells are getting powered and are healing(7 seconds pause)

155. Every day you wake up for a new start, a new journey(7 seconds pause)

156. You believe this process and have confidence in yourself(7 seconds pause)

157. You trust the journey(7 seconds pause)

158. You are confident enough(7 seconds pause)

159. You are generous towards yourself(7 seconds pause)
160. You enjoy your food and eat mindfully(7 seconds pause)
161. You chew slowly and enjoy the taste(7 seconds pause)
162. You are strong enough(7 seconds pause)
163. You deserve every bit of the love and care that you get(7 seconds pause)
164. You shed off sweat every day and take care of your body(7 seconds pause)
165. You are determined and full of courage(7 seconds pause)
166. You forgive for all the mistakes that you did unintentionally(7 seconds pause)
167. You like to stay mindful in the present(7 seconds pause)
168. You know how to ignore the feeling of emotional eating(7 seconds pause)
169. You are conscious of your eating schedule(7 seconds pause)
170. You have a daily goal of workout and eating healthy(7 seconds pause)
171. You stuff yourself only when you are starving(7 seconds pause)
172. You are enjoying this beautiful journey of walking on the path of being fit(7 seconds pause)
173. You enjoy each day of this journey(7 seconds pause)
174. You see the outcome soon(7 seconds pause)

175. You become more and more confident with each passing day(7 seconds pause)
176. You are getting fitter and slimmer(7 seconds pause)
177. You enjoy eating healthy(7 seconds pause)
178. You enjoy being in your body(7 seconds pause)
179. You consume food rich in nutrients(7 seconds pause)
180. You eat fruits and vegetables in different colors (7 seconds pause)
181. You can identify the difference between mental and physical hunger(7 seconds pause)
182. You choose food wisely(7 seconds pause)
183. You enjoy life to the fullest(7 seconds pause)
184. You are determined to achieve your goal weight(7 seconds pause)
185. You work out every day for half an hour(7 seconds pause)
186. The process encourages you when you notice it in the mirror(7 seconds pause)
187. You listen to the recordings most often and that helps you keep moving in this journey(7 seconds pause)
188. You have high self-confidence (7 seconds pause)
189. You are full of worth(7 seconds pause)
190. You are beautiful and amazing the way you are(7 seconds pause)
191. You are fitter than ever(7 seconds pause)

192. You are in good mood and give positive vibes always(7 seconds pause)
193. You are positive and joyful(7 seconds pause)
194. You like positive energy surrounding you(7 seconds pause)
195. You look at the glass half-full day-to-day(7 seconds pause)
196. You are thankful for this life and all the amazing things that you have(7 seconds pause)
197. Just by three breaths, you fall asleep as soon as you lie down o the bed(7 seconds pause(
198. When you press the index finger by the thumb you feel comfortable and calm(7 seconds pause)
199. You are becoming leaner and stronger(7 seconds pause)
200. You look amazingly beautiful(7 seconds pause)
201. You amazingly look after your body (7 seconds pause)
202. With every passing day you become fitter and healthier (7 seconds pause)
203. You love living every day (7 seconds pause)
204. You look forward to living a healthy lifestyle (7 seconds pause)
205. You are consciously eating (7 seconds pause)

206. You are mindful of your eating (7 seconds pause)
207. You love yourself unconditionally (7 seconds pause)
208. You are ready to transform yourself (7 seconds pause)
209. You achieve your daily goals (7 seconds pause)
210. You are mindful of your eating habits (7 seconds pause)
211. You sleep well (7 seconds pause)
212. You sleep on time and wake up fresh and happy (7 seconds pause)
213. Your days are brighter and happier (7 seconds pause)
214. You look healthy (7 seconds pause)
215. You enjoy healthy food (7 seconds pause)
216. You look happy (7 seconds pause)
217. You get compliments from friends and family (7 seconds pause)
218. You appreciate your efforts and your healthy body (7 seconds pause)
219. You eat healthy food (7 seconds pause)
220. You enjoy healthy eating (7 seconds pause)
221. You enjoy the sight and taste of green vegetables (7 seconds pause)
222. You love being healthy (7 seconds pause)
223. You are healthy (7 seconds pause)
224. Each organ is brimming with health and vitality (7 seconds pause)

225. You are attractive in every way (7 seconds pause)
226. You are smart and good enough (7 seconds pause)
227. You enjoy healthy foods (7 seconds pause)
228. Life is good (7 seconds pause) (7 seconds pause)
229. You enjoy your workouts (7 seconds pause)
230. You move your body more. (7 seconds pause)
231. Your body is getting sculpted with every passing day. (7 seconds pause)
232. Your body is more toned (7 seconds pause)
233. People appreciate your efforts (7 seconds pause)
234. You are inspiring (7 seconds pause)
235. You have inspired many already (7 seconds pause)
236. You enjoy living each day (7 seconds pause)
237. You are active (7 seconds pause)
238. You are fit (7 seconds pause)
239. You are positive (7 seconds pause)
240. You are happy (7 seconds pause)
241. You eat smaller portios of healthy food (7 seconds pause)
242. You have fast metabolism (7 seconds pause)
243. You enjoy the taste of fresh fruits and vegetables (7 seconds pause)

244. You drink atleast 8 to 10 glasses of water daily

245. You have a flat stomach

246. You fall asleep easily as soon as you get to the bed for the purpose of sleeping

247. You burn fat while sleeping

248. You are lovable

249. You are getting even more attractive

250. You forgive yourself for all the past mistakes

251. You also forgive others

252. You have high self esteem

253. You are confident

254. You are losing weight with every passing day

255. You are focused on your weight loss journey

256. You pay more attention to the journey than the ideal goal weight (7 seconds pause)

257. You are good enough (7 seconds pause)

258. You have high confidence (7 seconds pause)

259. You are an achiever (7 seconds pause)

260. You take pride in your achievements (7 seconds pause)

261. You eat only when you are physically hungry (7 seconds pause)

262. You do not eat when you are emotionally hungry(7 seconds pause)

263. You believe in yourself (7 seconds pause)
264. Your body is coming in shape (7 seconds pause)
265. You trust your body (7 seconds pause)
266. You trust yourself (7 seconds pause)
267. You trust the process of life (7 seconds pause)
268. You entire body is accepting the new weight loss regimen (7 seconds pause)
269. You are improving in every way , every day (7 seconds pause)
270. You are mindful of what you eat (7 seconds pause)
271. You enjoy your weight loss journey
272. You are the creator of your future. (7 seconds pause)
273. You are in a better space when it comes to food. (7 seconds pause)
274. The choices and decisions you make for yourself are for your higher good. (7 seconds pause)
275. You are no longer holding on to any regrets or guilt about your past food choices. (7 seconds pause)
276. You have accepted your body's shape and you feel blessed for what you have. (7 seconds pause)
277. You have moved away from toxic relationships (7 seconds pause)
278. You accept and acknowledge your strengths (7 seconds pause)

279. You allow yourself to feel good about being you. (7 seconds pause)
280. You have an acceptance for yourself. (7 seconds pause)
281. You are hopeful. (7 seconds pause)
282. You see your future filled with certainly and hope (7 seconds pause)
283. You think of your tropical island every time you decide to sleep 7 seconds pause)
284. Falling asleep is easier than you thought 7 seconds pause)
285. You enjoy your sleep time (7 seconds pause)
286. Your mind knows the importance of sleeping on time 7 seconds pause)
287. You maintain sleep hygiene (7 seconds pause)
288. You do not have caffeine post 5 pm (7 seconds pause)
289. You look forward to sleeping on time every night (7 seconds pause)
290. You are getting mentally stronger with every passing day (7 seconds pause)
291. Life is good with good healthy food and exercising habits 7 seconds pause)
292.
293. You enjoy your workouts 7 seconds pause)
294. You drink plenty of water 7 seconds pause)

CPSIA information can be obtained
at www.ICGtesting.com
Printed in the USA
BVHW081356120521
607050BV00008B/1889

9 781801 348195